# KETOGENIC DIET COOKBOOK

Low-Carb, High-Fat Recipes for Busy People on the Keto Diet

Amelia Wilson

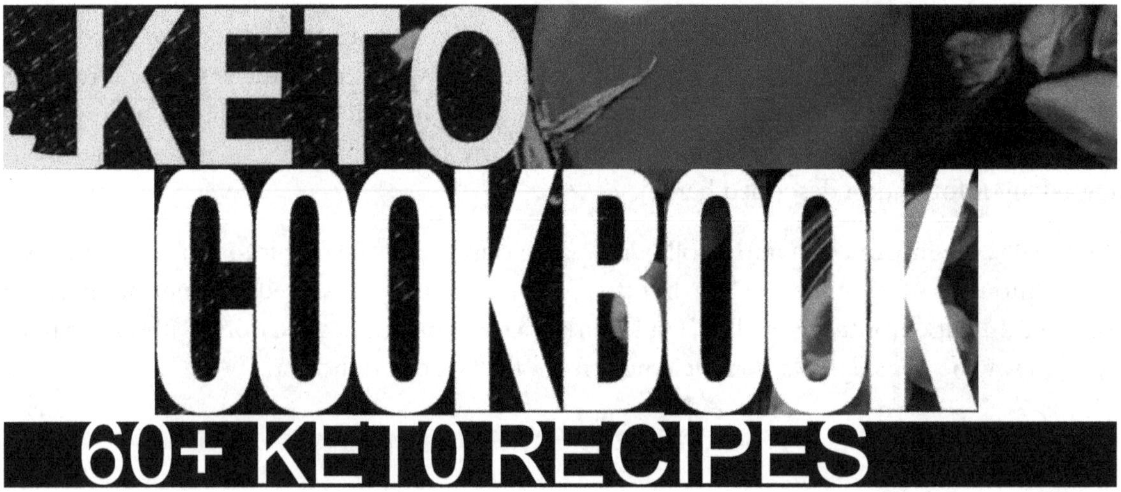
KETO
COOKBOOK
60+ KETO RECIPES

# TABLE OF CONTENTS

# BREAKFAST RECIPES

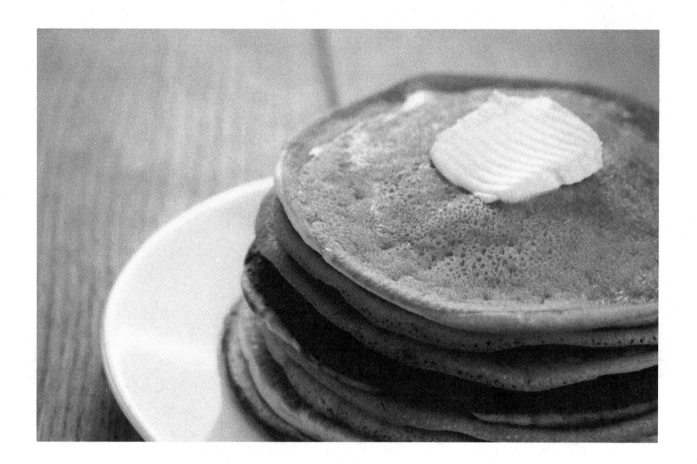

# KETO BREAKFAST MUFFINS

Serves:        *6-8*
Prep Time:     *10*   Minutes

Cook Time:     *15*   Minutes

Total Time:    *25*   Minutes

## INGREDIENTS

- 3 tablespoons plain Keto& Hot breakfast cereal
- 3 eggs
- 2 tablespoons heavy cream
- 2 tablespoons flaxseed meal
- 3 tablespoons coconut oil
- 2 tablespoons Erythritol
- 1 tsp vanilla extract
- 1 tsp baking powder

## DIRECTIONS

1. Preheat oven to 325 F
2. In a bowl mix Plain keto & Hot breakfast cereal, add coconut oil and mix well
3. Add the rest of ingredients and mix
4. Pour batter into 6-8 cupcakes and bake for 15-18 minutes
5. Remove and serve

# KETO PANCAKES

Serves: **4**

Prep Time: **10** Minutes

Cook Time: **10** Minutes

Total Time: **20** Minutes

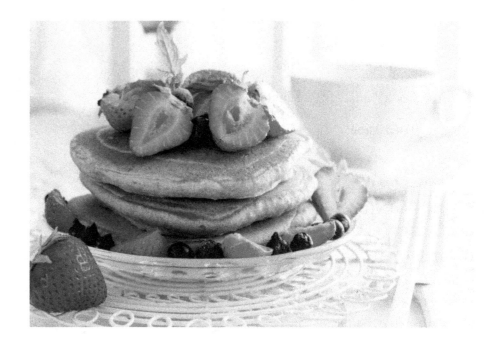

## INGREDIENTS

- **½ cup almond flour**
- **3 eggs**
- **½ tsp cinnamon**
- **1 tablespoon butter**
- **½ cup cream cheese**

## DIRECTIONS

1. **Place all ingredients in a bowl and mix using a blender**

2. **In a frying pan pour 2-3 tablespoons of pancake mixture and cook for 1-2 minutes per side**

3. **Remove and top with cinnamon or butter**

# BREAKFAST SANDWICH

Serves:       *1*
Prep Time:    *5*  Minutes

Cook Time:    *5*  Minutes

Total Time:  *10*  Minutes

## INGREDIENTS

- 3 tablespoons shredded cheddar cheese
- 1 egg
- 1 slice bacon
- Salt

## DIRECTIONS

1. In a skillet add shredded cheese oven medium heat
   and remove to a paper towel when it starts to melt

2. Cook the egg as you want, place it over the cheese and season with salt

3. Place the remaining cheese over the top and serve

# POWER BREAKFAST WITH GREEN SAUCE

Serves:      *3*

Prep Time:   *10*   Minutes

Cook Time:   *10*   Minutes

Total Time:  *20*   Minutes

## INGREDIENTS

- 1 cup baby spinach
- salt
- 1 cup parsley
- 4 garlic cloves
- 4 tablespoons hemp hearts
- 1 cup olive oil
- 4 slices bacon
- 1 cup arugula
- 1 egg
- 10 asparagus tips

## DIRECTIONS

1. For Green Sauce mix arugula, olive oil, parsley, garlic cloves, baby spinach, hemp hearts in a blender and blend until smooth

2. Arrange bacon sliced into rings and place the bacon in the oven at 325 F and cook until done

3. Tuck 3-4 asparagus tips into each bacon ring and add green sauce, sprinkle salt and pepper and cook for another 12-15 minutes

4. Remove from oven and serve

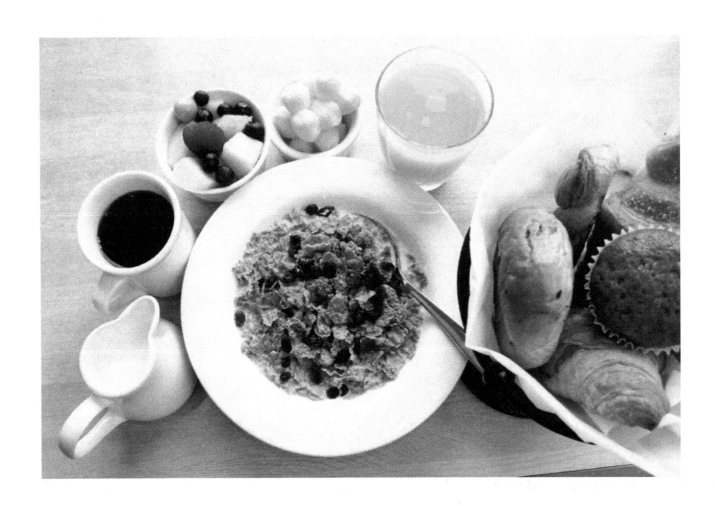

# PEPPER RINGS

Serves: **2**

Prep Time: **10** Minutes

Cook Time: **10** Minutes

Total Time: **20** Minutes

## INGREDIENTS

- 2 red bell peppers
- salt
- pepper
- 6 eggs
- 1 lb. breakfast sausage
- 3 tablespoons parmesan cheese
- coconut oil

## DIRECTIONS

1. In a skillet brown breakfast sausage and set aside
2. Cut peppers into 4-6 rings and place them in the skillet and cook
3. Pour the egg into the ring and add salt and sausage around the yolk of each ring
4. When ready remove and serve

# KETO EGG BITES

Serves:        *2*

Prep Time:    *10*  Minutes

Cook Time:    *20*  Minutes

Total Time:   *30*  Minutes

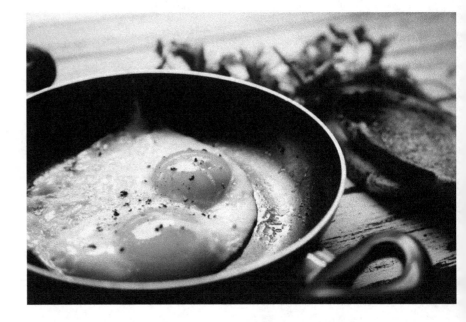

## INGREDIENTS

- 4 eggs
- ½ cup swiss cheese
- ½ cup fat cottage cheese
- ½ tsp salt
- black pepper
- 2 thick slices of paleo sugar free bacon

## DIRECTIONS

1. Preheat oven to 325 F and place a baking dish
2. In a bowl mix cottage cheese, salt, pepper cheese, eggs and blend until smooth
3. Spray a muffin tin and pour the mixture into it, add chopped bacon and bake for 25 minutes
4. Remove and serve

# BREAKFAST BOWL

Serves: *1*

Prep Time: *10* Minutes

Cook Time: *10* Minutes

Total Time: *20* Minutes

## INGREDIENTS

- 2 eggs
- 2 strips bacon
- ½ up cheddar cheese
- ½ cup salsa
- 2 tablespoons butter
- ½ avocado

## DIRECTIONS

1. In a bowl scramble the eggs and place them into the skillet, cook for 2-3 minutes
2. Top the eggs with shredded cheese and bacon
3. Slice avocado and place it over the bacon
4. Top with salsa and serve

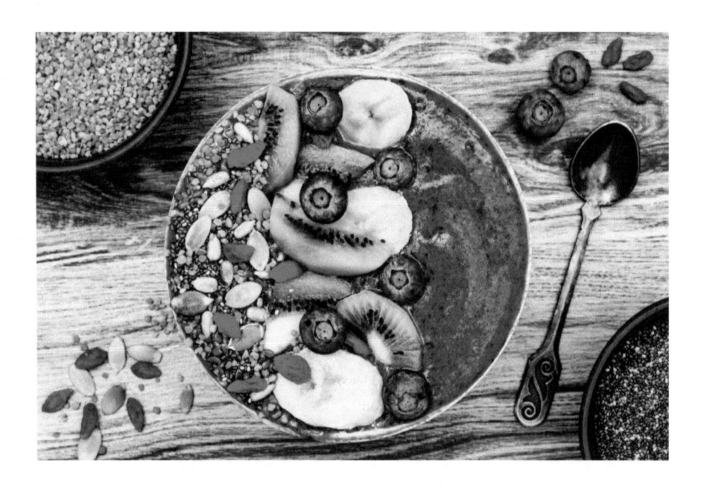

# KETO POTATOES

Serves: **4**

Prep Time: **10** Minutes

Cook Time: **10** Minutes

Total Time: **20** Minutes

## INGREDIENTS

- 1 large turnip
- ½ paprika, garlic powder, salt
- parsley
- ½ onion
- 2 slices bacon
- 1 tablespoon olive oil

## DIRECTIONS

1. In a skillet add the turnips and spices, cook for 5-6 minutes, add onion and cook for another 2-3 minutes

2. Chop the bacon and add to the skillet, cook for another 2-3 minutes

3. Remove to a place and top with parsley before serving

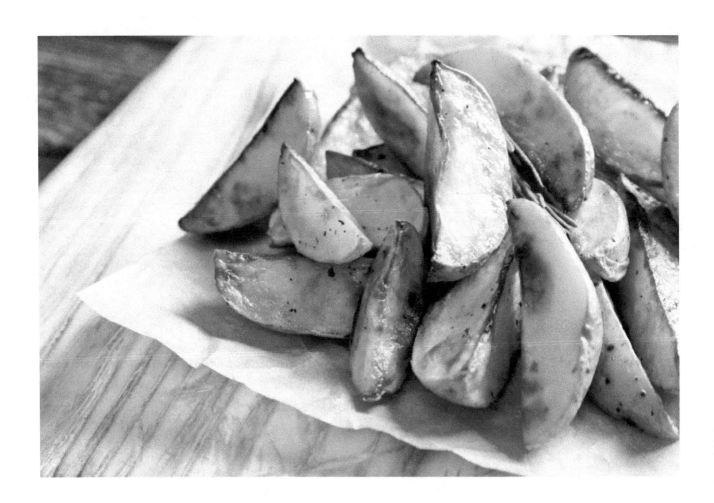

# MINI BREAKFAST MEATLOAFS

Serves:        **4**

Prep Time:   **10**   Minutes

Cook Time:   **30**   Minutes

Total Time:  **40**   Minutes

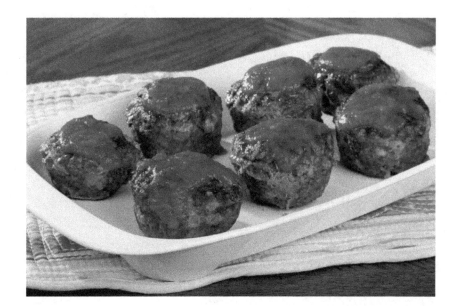

### INGREDIENTS

- 1 lb. pork sausage
- 1 egg
- 1 cup shredded cheddar cheese
- 4 slices bacon
- 4 slices ham

### DIRECTIONS

1. Preheat oven to 325 F
2. In a bowl mix all ingredients
3. Divide mixture into 6-8 portions and pack into mini loaf pan cavities
4. Bake for 30 minutes, remove and serve

# KETO JALAPENO MUFFINS

Serves:        *4*
Prep Time:    *10*  Minutes
Cook Time:    *30*  Minutes
Total Time:   *40*  Minutes

## INGREDIENTS

- 8 eggs
- 8 oz. cheese
- ¾ cup heavy cream
- salt
- jalapeno
- 8 slices bacon

## DIRECTIONS

1. Preheat oven to 325
2. Add bacon to each muffin tin
3. In a bowl mix cream, cheese, pepper, eggs and salt
4. Distribute into 8-10 muffin cups and add jalapeno to each muffin tin
5. Bake for 15-20 minutes, when ready remove and serve

# *LUNCH RECIPES*

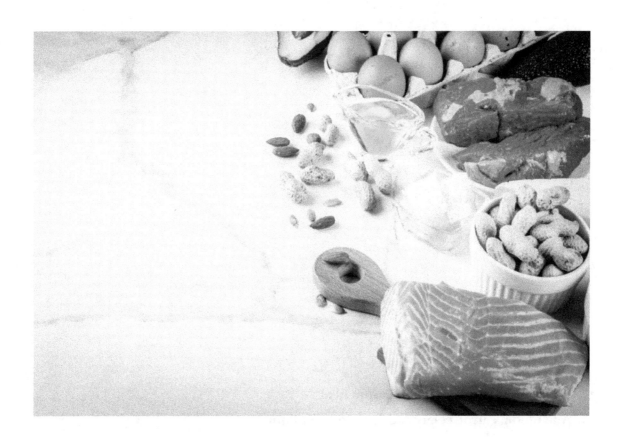

# SOUP RECIPES KETO BROCCOLI SOUP

Serves: **4**

Prep Time: **10** Minutes

Cook Time: **30** Minutes

Total Time: **40** Minutes

## INGREDIENTS

- olive oil
- 1 cup chicken broth
- 1 cup heavy whipping cream
- 6 oz. shredded cheddar cheese
- salt
- 5-ounces broccoli
- 1 celery stalk
- 1 small carrot
- ½ onion

## DIRECTIONS

1. In a pot add olive oil over medium heat
2. Add onion, carrot, celery and cook for 2-3 minutes
3. Add chicken broth and simmer for 4-5 minutes
4. Stir in broccoli and cream
5. Sprinkle in cheese and season with salt

# KETO TACO SOUP

Serves:        *8*
Prep Time:    *10*  Minutes
Cook Time:    *10*  Minutes
Total Time:   *20*  Minutes

## INGREDIENTS

- 2 lbs. ground beef
- 1 onion
- 1 cup heavy whipping cream
- 1 tsp chili powder
- 14 oz. cream cheese
- 1 tsp garlic
- 1 tsp cumin
- 2 10 oz. cans tomatoes
- 16 oz. beef broth

## DIRECTIONS

1. Cook for a couple of minutes, onion, garlic and beef
2. Add cream cheese and stir until fully melted
3. Add tomatoes, whipping cream, beef broth, stir and bring to boil

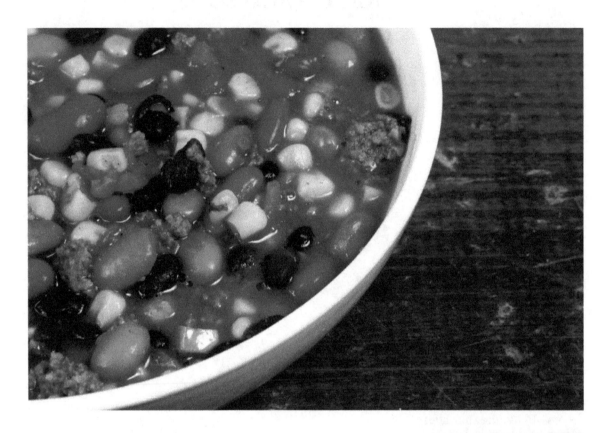

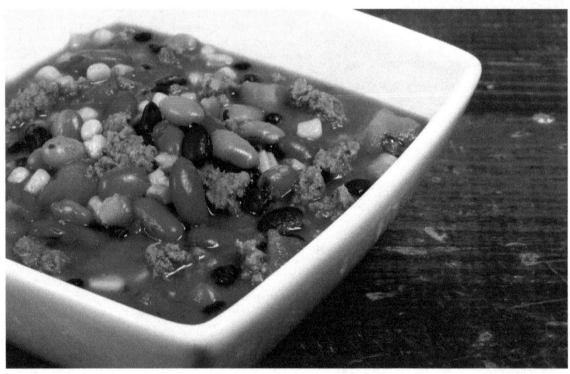

# KETO CHICKEN SOUP

Serves:        **4**
Prep Time:   **10**  Minutes
Cook Time:   **30**  Minutes
Total Time:  **40**  Minutes

## INGREDIENTS

- 2 boneless chicken breast
- 20-ounces  diced tomatoes
- ½ tsp salt
- 1 cup salsa
- 6-ounces cream cheese
- avocado
- 2 tablespoons taco seasoning
- 1 cup chicken broth

## DIRECTIONS

1. In a slow cooker place all ingredients and cook for 5-6 hours or until chicken is tender
2. Whisk cream cheese into the broth
3. When ready, remove and serve

# KETO SPINACH SOUP

Serves:          **2**
Prep Time:    **5**   Minutes
Cook Time:   **15**   Minutes
Total Time:   **20**   Minutes

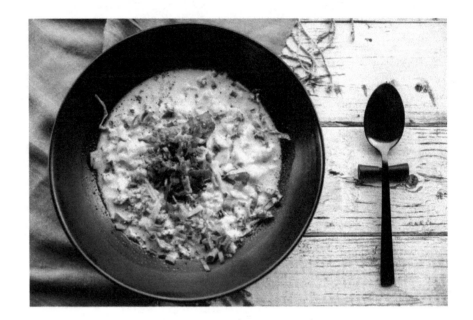

## INGREDIENTS

- ¼ lbs. spinach
- 2 oz. onion
- ¼ lbs. heavy cream
- ½ oz. garlic
- 1 chicken stock cube
- 1,5 cup water
- 1 tablespoons butter

## DIRECTIONS

1. In a saucepan melt the butter and sauté the onion
2. Add garlic, spinach and stock cube and half the water
3. Cook until spinach wilts
4. Pour everything in a blender and blend, add water
5. Serve with pepper and toasted nuts

# KETO TOSCANA SOUP

Serves:         **4**
Prep Time:   **10**   Minutes
Cook Time:  **30**   Minutes
Total Time:  **40**   Minutes

## INGREDIENTS

- 1 lb. Italian sausage
- ½ cup whipping cream
- 1 tsp garlic
- 2 cup kale leaves
- 1 bag radishes 16-ounces
- 1 onion
- 30-ounces vegetable broth

## DIRECTIONS

1. Cut radishes into small chunks and blend until smooth
2. In a pot add onion and sausage, cook until brown, add radishes, broth
3. Cook on medium heat, add heavy whipping cream, kale leaves
4. Cook for a couple minutes
5. Remove and serve

# KETO PARMESAN SOUP

Serves: **4**

Prep Time: **10** Minutes

Cook Time: **30** Minutes

Total Time: **40** Minutes

## INGREDIENTS

- 1 broccoli
- 1 tsp pepper
- 1 tablespoon butter
- 1 tablespoon cheese
- 1 onion
- ½ cup warm
- 1 tsp salt
- ½ cup heavy cream

## DIRECTIONS

1. In a saucepan add onion and cook
2. Stir in broccoli and cook until soft
3. Combine with heavy cream and place in a blender, blend until smooth
4. Return the soup to the saucepan, season with salt
5. Serve and sprinkle with parmesan

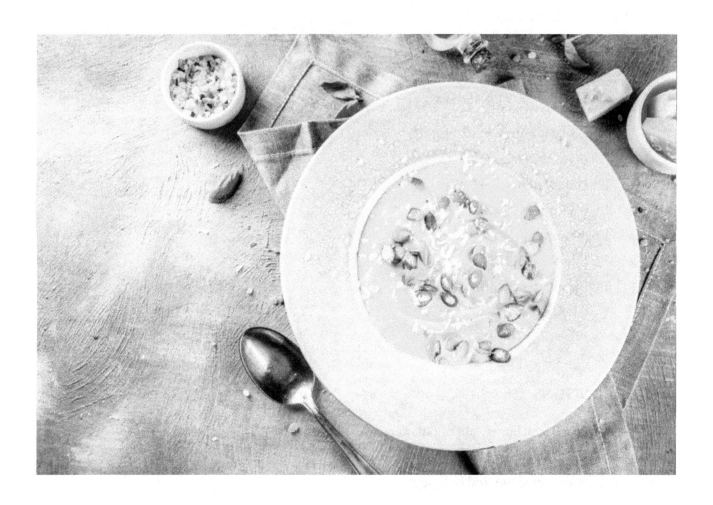

# KETO CAULIFLOWER SOUP

Serves: **4**

Prep Time: **10** Minutes

Cook Time: **30** Minutes

Total Time: **40** Minutes

## INGREDIENTS

- ½ head of cauliflower
- ½ cup heavy cream
- ½ red bell pepper
- 1 tsp salt
- 1 tsp pepper
- 1 tablespoon butter
- 1 tablespoons parmesan cheese
- 1 tsp herbs

## DIRECTIONS

1. In a saucepan melt butter, add cauliflower and cook **until soft**
2. Remove from saucepan and set aside
3. Melt butter and sauté and bell pepper
4. In a food processor add cauliflower mixture, pepper and cook for 4-5 minutes
5. Season with salt and pepper
6. Garnish with parmesan and serve

# KETO BROCCOLI CHEESE SOUP

Serves: **2**

Prep Time: **10** Minutes

Cook Time: **20** Minutes

Total Time: **30** Minutes

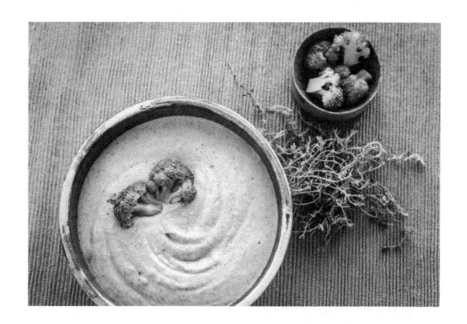

## INGREDIENTS

- 2 cups broccoli
- 3 cups chicken broth
- 1 onion
- 1 cup heavy cream
- 6 oz. cream cheese
- 1 tablespoon hot sauce
- 3 tablespoons butter
- 1 clove garlic
- 6 oz. cheddar cheese

## DIRECTIONS

1. In a saucepan melt butter, add onion, garlic and sauté until soft
2. Pour in heavy cream, chicken broth, stir in broccoli
3. Cover and continue cooking for 12-15 minutes
4. Add cheese and cook until melted
5. Stir in hot sauce and enjoy

# KETO QUESO SOUP

Serves:       **4**

Prep Time:    **10**  Minutes

Cook Time:    **30**  Minutes

Total Time:   **40**  Minutes

## INGREDIENTS

- 1 lb. chicken breast
- 1 tablespoon taco seasoning
- 1 tablespoon avocado oil
- 1 can diced green chilies
- 6-ounces cream cheese
- ½ cup heavy cream
- salt
- 2 cups chicken broth

## DIRECTIONS

1. In an iron Dutch oven heat oil over medium heat stir in taco seasoning and cook for 1-2 minutes

2. Add broth, chicken and simmer for 20 minutes, remove chicken and shred

3. Stir in cream cheese and heavy cream into the soup, once the cheese has melted, add the chicken back to the soup, season with salt and serve

# KETO CRAB SOUP

Serves:          **6**
Prep Time:    **10**  Minutes
Cook Time:   **10**  Minutes
Total Time:   **20**  Minutes

## INGREDIENTS

- 1 tablespoon butter
- 1 tablespoon seasoning
- 6-ounces cream cheese
- ¾ cup parmesan cheese
- 1 lb. lump crabmeat

## DIRECTIONS

1. In a pot melt butter and add seasoning, cream cheese and whisk until smooth
2. Add parmesan cheese, crab meat and reduce heat
3. Simmer until is done
4. Remove and serve

# <u>*SALAD*</u>

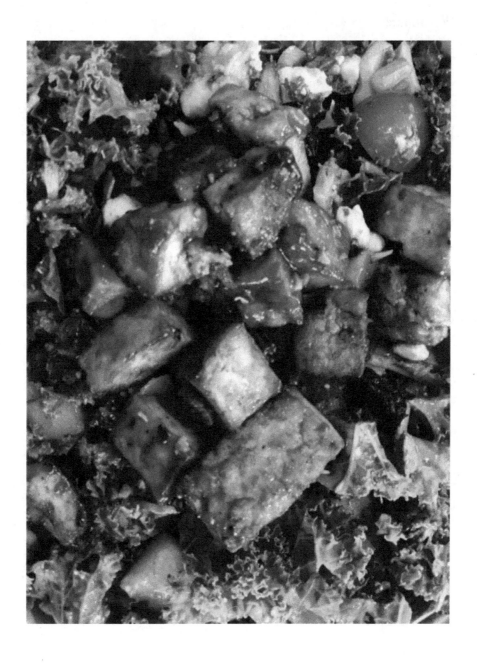

# KETO SALAD

Serves: **2**

Prep Time: **10** Minutes

Cook Time: **10** Minutes

Total Time: **20** Minutes

## INGREDIENTS

- 1 slice bacon
- 3-ounces chicken breast
- 1-ounce cheddar cheese
- 1 tablespoon olive oil
- 1 tablespoon apple cider vinegar
- ½ avocado
- 1 head romaine lettuce

## DIRECTIONS

1. Chop all ingredients and place them in a bowl
2. Mix well and add pepper, oil and vinegar

# KETO BROCCOLI SALAD

Serves: **2**

Prep Time: **10** Minutes

Cook Time: **10** Minutes

Total Time: **20** Minutes

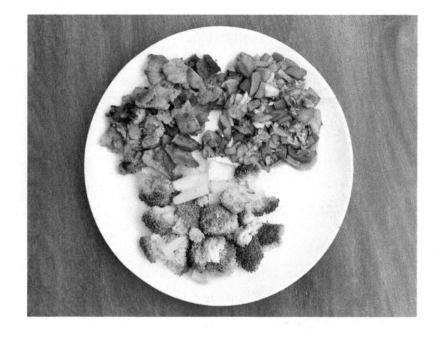

## INGREDIENTS

- 20-ounce raw broccoli
- 1 cup bacon
- ½ red onion
- 1 cup avocado mayo
- 1 cup macadamia nuts
- ½ cup Monkfruit sweetener
- 1 tablespoon organic apple cider vinegar

## DIRECTIONS

1. Place Macadamia Nuts in a blender and blend until smooth
2. Place all ingredients in a bowl and mix well, pour over Macadamia Nuts mixture and serve

# KETO GREEN SPRING SALAD

Serves: **4**

Prep Time: **10** Minutes

Cook Time: **30** Minutes

Total Time: **40** Minutes

## INGREDIENTS

- 2-ounces mixed greens
- 2 tablespoons pine nuts
- 1 tablespoon raspberry vinaigrette
- 1 tablespoon parmesan
- 1 slice bacon
- salt and pepper

## DIRECTIONS

1. Cook bacon until crispy
2. Place greens in a bowl with the rest of ingredients
3. Top with bacon and serve

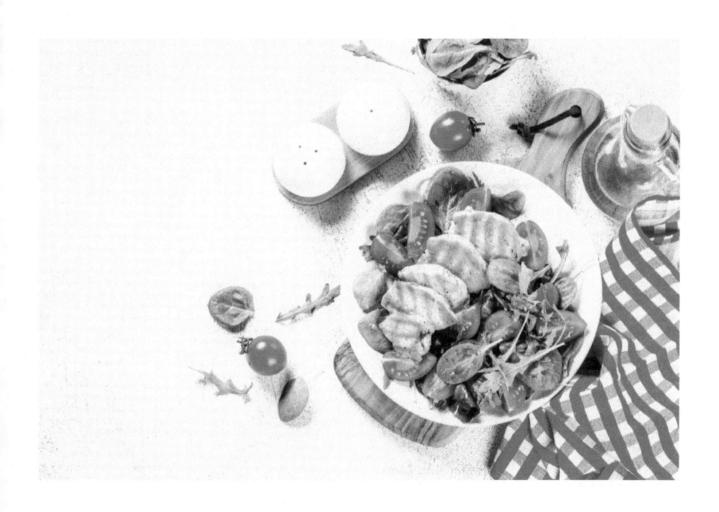

# KETO EGG SALAD

Serves: **4**

Prep Time: **10** Minutes

Cook Time: **30** Minutes

Total Time: **40** Minutes

## INGREDIENTS

- 6 eggs
- 2 celery stalks
- 2 green onion stalks
- 1 green pepper
- 1 tsp mustard
- 2/3 cup mayonnaise

## DIRECTIONS

1. Hard boil eggs and remove to a bowl
2. Chop green pepper, onions and celery
3. In a bowl mix all the ingredients and serve

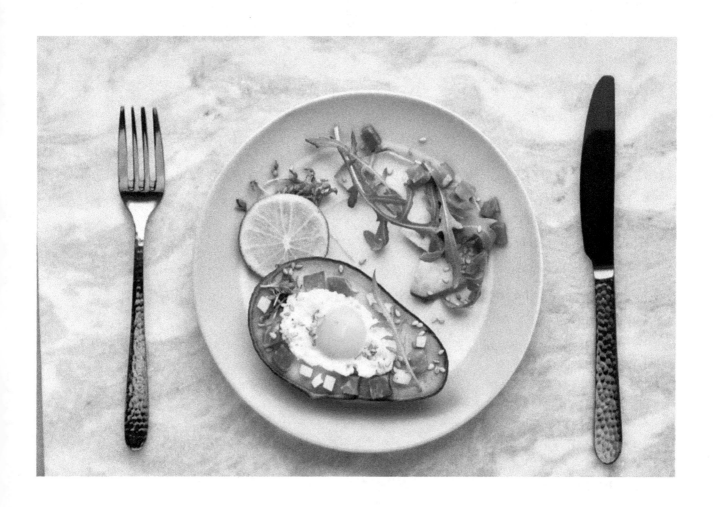

# KETO CAESAR SALAD

Serves:        *4*

Prep Time:   *10*  Minutes

Cook Time:  *30*  Minutes

Total Time:  *40*  Minutes

## INGREDIENTS

- 10 oz. chicken breasts
- 1 tablespoon olive oil
- salt
- 2 oz. bacon
- 6 oz. romaine lettuce
- 1 oz. parmesan cheese **DRESSING**
- ½ cup mayonnaise
- 1 tablespoon chopped filets of anchovies
- 1 garlic clove
- 1 tablespoon mustard
- ½ lemon zest
- 1 tablespoon parmesan cheese

## DIRECTIONS

1. In a bowl mix all ingredients for the dressing and set aside
2. Preheat oven to 400 F and place chicken breast in a baking dish and bake for 15-20 minutes
3. In a bowl place sliced chicken, all the salad ingredients, dressing and mix well
4. Serve with parmesan cheese

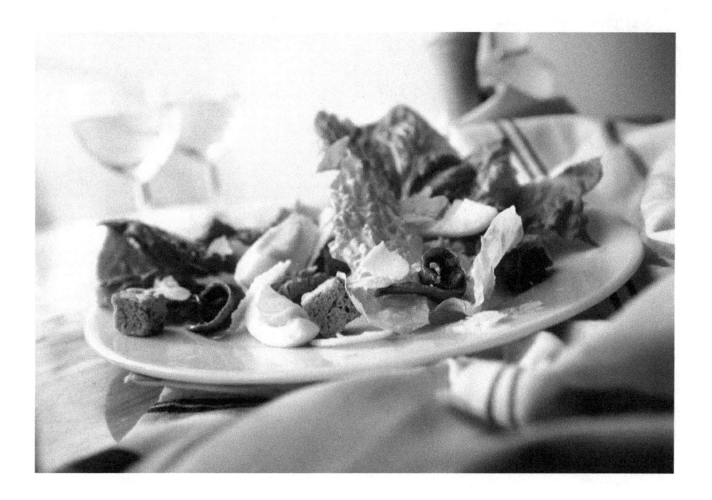

# KETO PEPPERONI SALAD

Serves: **4**
Prep Time: **10** Minutes
Cook Time: **30** Minutes
Total Time: **40** Minutes

## INGREDIENTS

- ½ avocado
- 12 slices pepperoni
- 1 oz. Mozzarella pears
- Italian seasoning

## DIRECTIONS

1. In a bowl mix all ingredients and serve

# KETO CHICKEN SALAD

Serves: **4**

Prep Time: **10** Minutes

Cook Time: **30** Minutes

Total Time: **40** Minutes

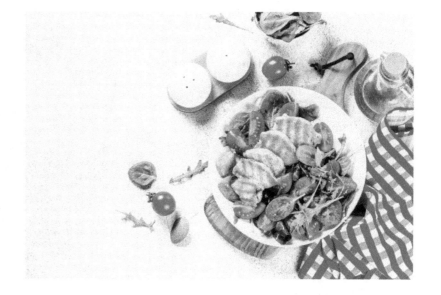

## INGREDIENTS

- 2 ribs celery
- ½ tsp pink Himalayan
- 1 tsp fresh dill
- ½ cup pecans
- 1 lb. chicken breast
- ½ cup mayo
- 1 tsp mustard

## DIRECTIONS

1. Preheat oven to 425 F and bake chicken breast for 15- 20 minutes
2. Remove chicken and cut into small pieces
3. In a bowl mix all ingredients and toss until chicken is fully coated
4. When ready, add dill and serve

# KETO TUNA SALAD

Serves: **4**

Prep Time: **10** Minutes

Cook Time: **30** Minutes

Total Time: **40** Minutes

## INGREDIENTS

- **1 can tuna**
- **½ tsp dill**
- **1 boiled egg**
- **1 slice bacon**
- **1 tablespoon mayo**
- **1 tablespoon sour cream**
- **1 tsp mustard**
- **1 tablespoon onion**

## DIRECTIONS

1. Prepare bacon, onion and boil egg
2. In a bowl place tuna, add egg and onion and the rest of ingredients
3. Top with bacon and serve

# SPINACH SALAD

Serves:        *4*
Prep Time:   *10*   Minutes
Cook Time:   *30*   Minutes
Total Time:  *40*   Minutes

## INGREDIENTS

- 2 cups spinach
- ½ avocado
- 1 strawberry **DRESSING**
- 2 slices bacon
- 1 tablespoon avocado oil
- pinch red pepper flakes
- 1 tsp oregano
- ½ tsp garlic powder
- ½ tsp salt
- half lemon

## DIRECTIONS

1. In a bowl mix all dressing ingredients
2. In another bowl mix salad ingredients and pour dressing over
3. Mix well and serve

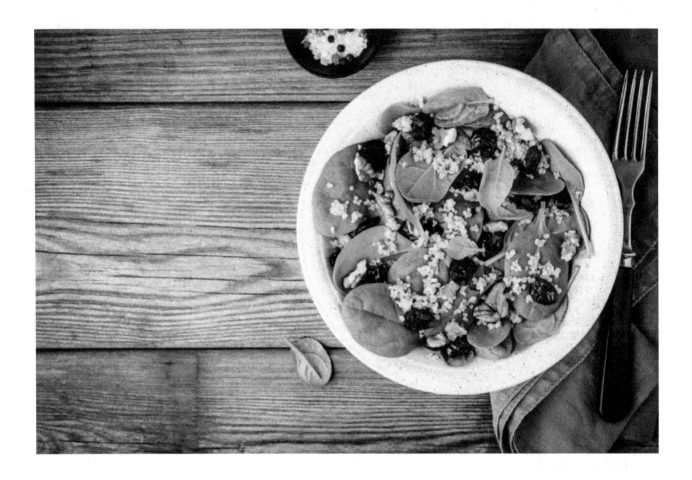

# KETO POTOTO SALAD

Serves:        *1*
Prep Time:     *10*  Minutes
Cook Time:     *10*  Minutes

Total Time:    *20*  Minutes

## INGREDIENTS

- 1 cauliflower
- 1 tablespoon mustard
- 1 tsp celery seeds
- ½ tsp salt
- ½ cup celery
- 1 tsp dill
- ½ cup sour cream
- ½ cup mayonnaise
- 2 stalks green onions
- 2 hard boiled eggs
- 1 tablespoon white vinegar

## DIRECTIONS

1. In a bowl prepare dressing by whisking together sour cream, celery seed, salt, mayonnaise, vinegar and mustard
2. In another bowl mix salad ingredient, pour dressing and mix well

# DINNER RECIPES

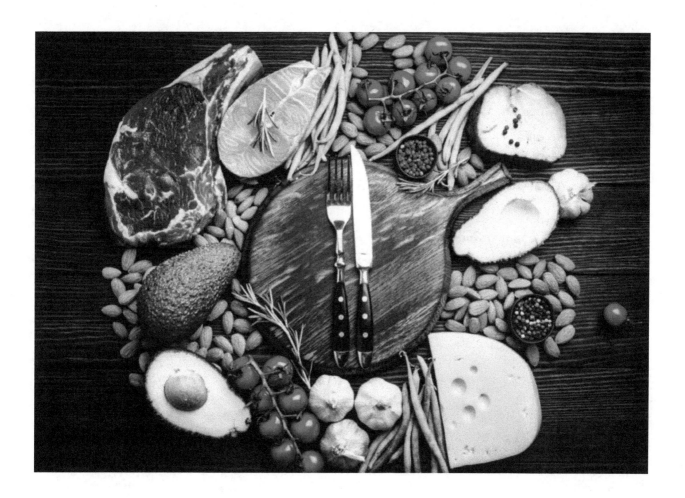

# KETO MONGOLAIN BEEF

Serves: **2**
Prep Time: **10** Minutes

Cook Time: **10** Minutes

Total Time: **20** Minutes

## INGREDIENTS

- 1 lb. flat iron steak
- ½ cup coconut oil
- 2 green onions

## LOW CARB MONGOLIAN BEEF MARINADE

- ½ cup coconut aminos
- 1 tsp ginger
- 1 clove garlic

## DIRECTIONS

1. Cut the flat iron steak into thin slices
2. Add the beef to a ziplock bag and add coconut aminos, garlic and ginger, marinate for 1 hour
3. Add coconut oil to a wok and cook beef on high heat for 2-3 minutes
4. Add green onions, cook for another 1-2 minutes
5. Remove and serve

# PEPPERONI KETO PIZZA

Serves:          *2*
Prep Time:   *10*   Minutes

Cook Time:   *10*   Minutes

Total Time:   *20*   Minutes

## INGREDIENTS

- 1 cauli'flour foods crust
- 2 oz. pepperoni
- ½ cup pizza sauce
- salt
- 2-ounces fresh mozzarella
- ½ cup jalapeno

## DIRECTIONS

1. Preheat oven to 375 F and place pizza crust on a vented pizza pan, cook for 8-10 minutes
2. Add mozzarella, sauce, pepperoni and jalapeno
3. Place back in the oven for 5-6 minutes
4. Remove and serve

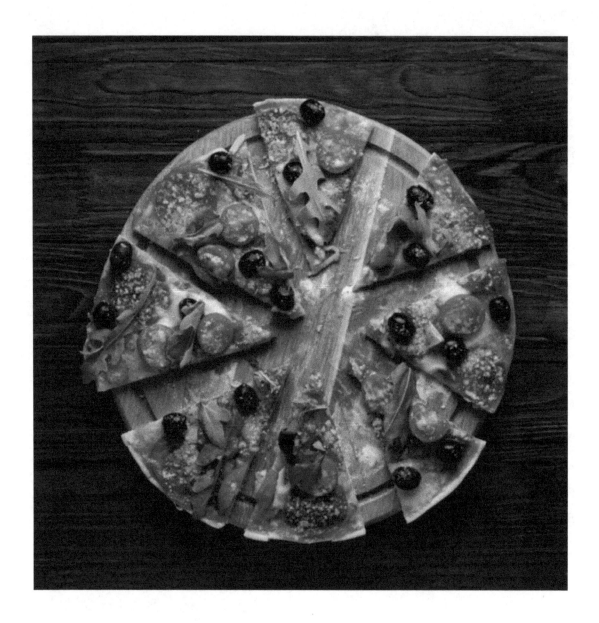

# QUICK KETO PIZZA

Serves: **4**

Prep Time: **10** Minutes

Cook Time: **10** Minutes

Total Time: **10** Minutes

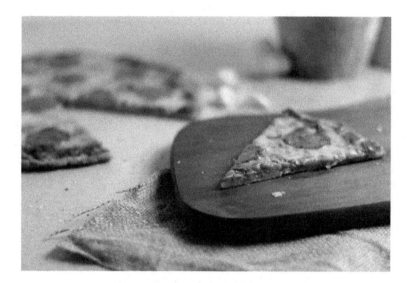

## INGREDIENTS

### PIZZA CRUST

- 2 eggs
- 1 tablespoon parmesan cheese
- 1 tablespoon husk powder
- ½ tsp Italian seasoning
- Salt

-2 tsp frying oil **TOPPINGS**

- 1 oz. mozzarella cheese
- 2 tablespoons. Tomato sauce
- 1 tablespoon chopped basil

## DIRECTIONS

1. In a bowl mix all pizza crust ingredients

2. Spoon the mixture into a pan, cook for 1 minute per side

3. Add cheese, tomato sauce and broil for 1-2 minutes **until cheese is bubbling**

# MUSHROOMS PIZZA

Serves:          *2*
Prep Time:    *10*   Minutes
Cook Time:    *15*   Minutes

Total Time:    *25*   Minutes

## INGREDIENTS

- ¼ cup rao's marinara
- pepperoni
- sliced baby bella mushrooms
- sliced ripe olives
- mozzarella

## DIRECTIONS

1. Preheat oven to 375 F
2. Spray a pie plate with a non-stick cooking spray
3. Spread marinara on bottom of pie plate
4. Layer mushrooms, pepperoni, olives and top with **mozzarella**
5. Bake for 10 minutes and serve

# BUFFALO KETO CHICKEN TENDERS

Serves: **2**

Prep Time: **10** Minutes

Cook Time: **30** Minutes

Total Time: **40** Minutes

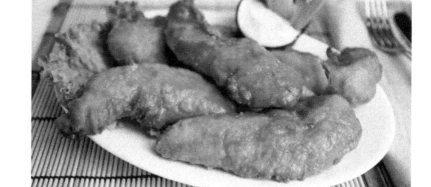

## INGREDIENTS

- 1 lb. chicken breast tenders
- 1 cup almond flour
- 1 egg
- 1 tablespoon heavy whipping cream
- 5 oz. buffalo sauce
- Salt

## DIRECTIONS

1. Preheat oven to 325 F
2. Season chicken with salt, pepper and almond flour
3. Beat 1 egg with heavy cream
4. Dip each tender in the egg and then into seasoned almond flour
5. Place tenders on a baking sheet and bake for 25 minutes or until crispy
6. Remove and serve

# KETO LASAGNA

Serves:         *4*
Prep Time:      *10*   Minutes

Cook Time:      *30*   Minutes

Total Time:     *40*   Minutes

## INGREDIENTS

- 1 lb. ground beef
- 1 cup sauce
- ¾ cup mozzarella
- 6 tablespoons ricotta
- salt, onion powder, Italian seasoning

## DIRECTIONS

1. Preheat oven to 350 F, brown beef and season
2. Being to layer a deep dish with noodle, ricotta, sauce mix and sprinkle with mozzarella, top with cheese
3. Bake for 20-25 minutes
4. Remove and serve

# KETO PARMESAN CASSEROLE

Serves: *3*

Prep Time: *10* Minutes

Cook Time: *30* Minutes

Total Time: *40* Minutes

## INGREDIENTS

- 2 cups cooked chicken
- ½ tsp basil
- 1 slice bacon
- ½ cup marinara sauce
- ½ tsp red pepper flakes
- ¾ cup mozzarella cheese
- ½ cup Parmesan cheese

## DIRECTIONS

1. Preheat the oven to 325 F
2. Lay out the chicken in the pan and spread the marinara sauce all over
3. Dredge the top with parmesan, red pepper flakes, mozzarella and sprinkle bacon and basil
4. Bake for 20-25 minutes, remove and serve

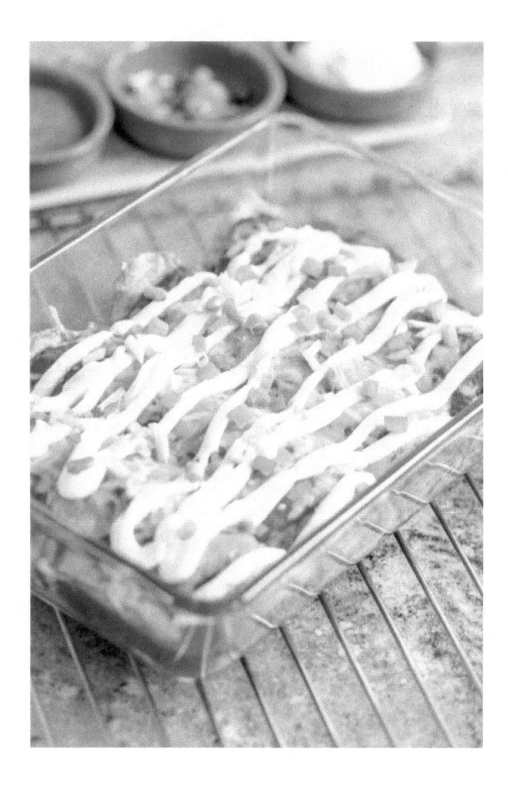

# KETO CHEESE MEATBALLS

Serves:        *2*

Prep Time:   *10*  Minutes

Cook Time:   *10*  Minutes

Total Time:  *20*  Minutes

## INGREDIENTS

- ½ lbs. beef mince
- 2 tablespoons parmesan cheese
- ½ tsp salt
- ½ tsp pepper
- ¼ lbs. cheese
- 1 tsp garlic powder

## DIRECTIONS

1. Cut the cheese into cubes
2. Mix all dry ingredients with the ground beef
3. Wrap the cubes of cheese in mince and pan fry the meatballs

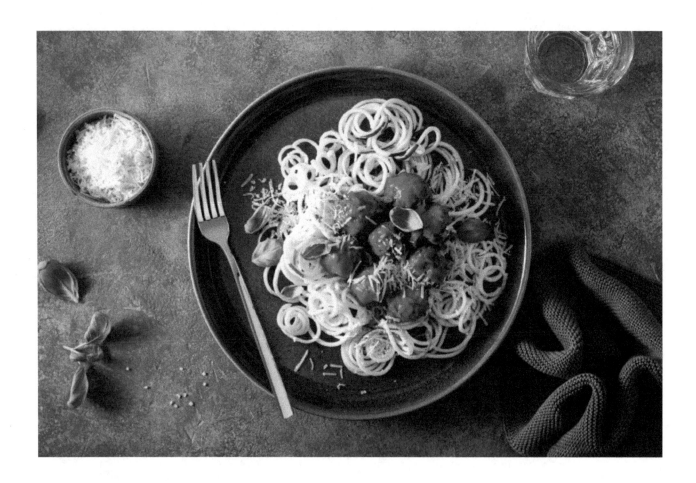

# KETO CHEESY BACON CHICKEN

Serves:          **4**

Prep Time:    **10**    Minutes

Cook Time:    **30**    Minutes

Total Time:    **40**    Minutes

## INGREDIENTS

- 5 chicken breasts
- 2 tablespoons seasoning rub
- ½ lbs. bacon
- 3 oz. shredded cheddar
- barbecue sauce

## DIRECTIONS

1. Preheat oven to 375 F and spray a baking sheet with cooking spray
2. Rub both sides of chicken breast with seasoning rub and top with bacon, bake for 25 minutes
3. Remove from oven, sprinkle with cheese and serve

# KETO CHEESEBURGER

Serves:        **2**
Prep Time:    **10**  Minutes
Cook Time:    **60**  Minutes
Total Time:   **70**  Minutes

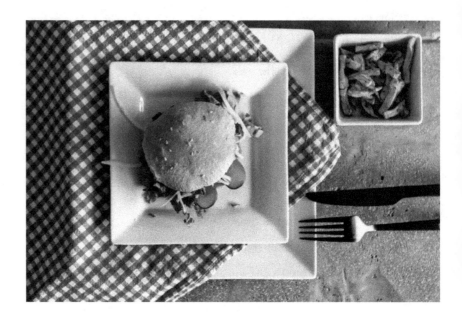

## INGREDIENTS

- 2 lbs. ground beef
- 2 eggs
- ½ cup grated parmesan
- 1 small onion
- 1 tsp salt
- 1 tsp garlic powder
- ½ cup cheddar cheese

## DIRECTIONS

1. In a bowl mix all ingredients except cheddar cheese, **add the end add cheese cubes**
2. Place mixture into a sprayed oven dish and form a **meatloaf shape**
3. Bake at 325 F for 50 minutes
4. Remove and serve

# DESSERT RECIPES

CAKE

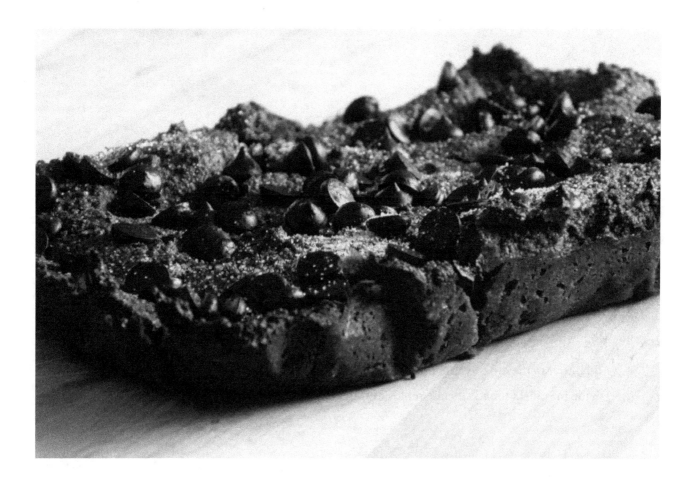

# CHEESECAKE KETO FAT BOMBS

Serves:       *12*

Prep Time:   *10*  Minutes

Cook Time:  *10*  Minutes

Total Time:  *20*  Minutes

## INGREDIENTS

- 5 oz. cream cheese
- 2 oz. frozen strawberries
- 2 oz. butter
- 1 oz. swerve sweetener
- 1 tsp vanilla extract

## DIRECTIONS

1. Puree the strawberries using a blender
2. In a bowl mix sweetener, vanilla, pureed strawberries and mix well
3. Microwave cream cheese and combine with the rest of **ingredients**
4. Add butter to the mixture and mix with an electric mixer
5. Divide into 10-12 round silicone molds and freeze for **1-2 hours before serving**

# KETO BROWNIES

Serves: **12**

Prep Time: **10** Minutes

Cook Time: **20** Minutes

Total Time: **30** Minutes

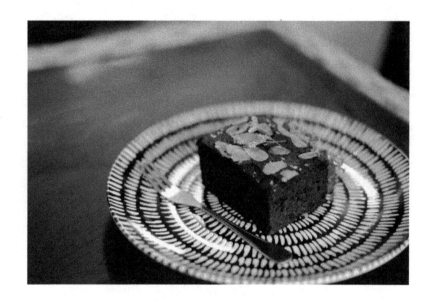

## INGREDIENTS

- ½ cup almond flour
- ½ tsp baking powder
- 1 tablespoon instant coffee
- 2 oz. chocolate
- 1 egg
- ½ tsp vanilla extract
- ½ cup cacao powder
- 2/3 cup Erythritol
- 8 tablespoons utter

## DIRECTIONS

1. Preheat oven to 325 F
2. In a medium bowl whisk almond flour, baking powder, Erythritol, cocoa powder and instant coffee
3. In another bowl melt chocolate and butter and whisk in the eggs and vanilla
4. Add to dry ingredients and mix well
5. Transfer batter into baking dish and bake for 20 minutes
6. Remove and serve

# KETO ICE CREAM

Serves:          *2*

Prep Time:    *10*   Minutes

Cook Time:   *20*   Minutes

Total Time:   *30*   Minutes

## INGREDIENTS

- 2 cups heavy cream
- 1 tablespoon milk powder
- ½ tsp xanthum gum
- 1 tsp vanilla extract
- 1 cup whole milk
- ½ cup truvia baking blend

## DIRECTIONS

1. In a bowl mix milk powder, sweetener, xanthum gum
2. Pour in cream, vanilla extract, milk and mix until sweetener is dissolved
3. Pour into ice cream maker and churn until set
4. Serve when ready

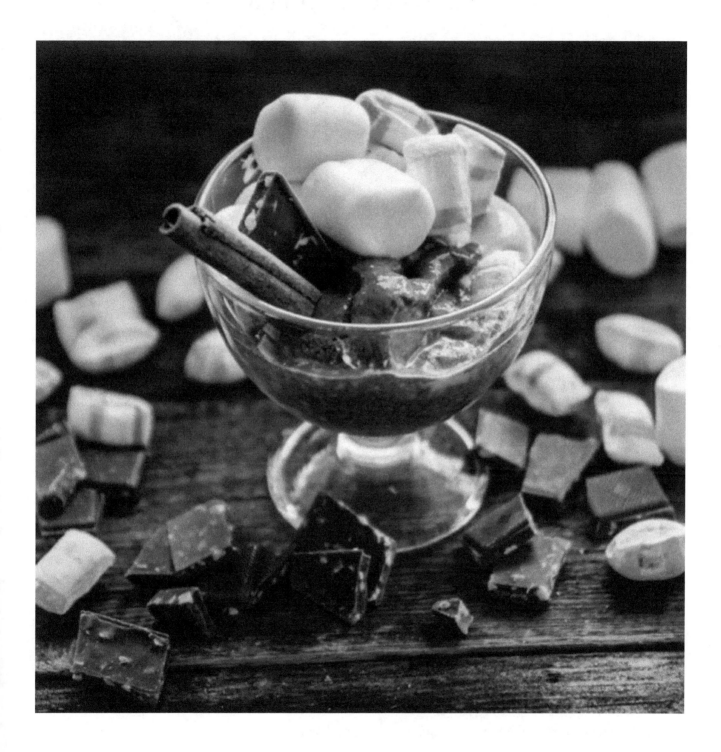

# KETO EGG CREPES

Serves: **2**

Prep Time: **10** Minutes

Cook Time: **10** Minutes

Total Time: **20** Minutes

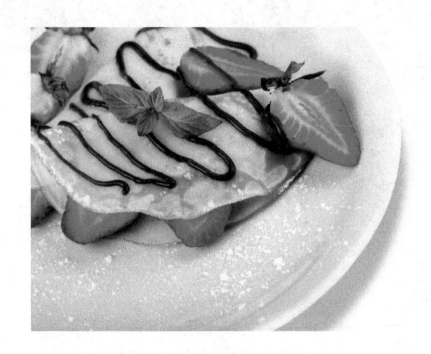

## INGREDIENTS

- 5 eggs
- 5 oz. cream cheese
- 1 tsp cinnamon
- 1 tablespoon sugar substitute
- butter FILLING
- 7 tablespoons butter
- ½ cup sugar substitute
- 1 tablespoon cinnamon

## DIRECTIONS

1. Blend all of the crepe ingredients until smooth
2. Pour batter into the pan and cook 1-2 minutes per side
3. Remove and pour mixture over the crepes
4. For crepes mixture mix cinnamon and sweetener in a bowl
5. Serve when ready

# KETO NAAN

Serves: **4**

Prep Time: **10** Minutes

Cook Time: **30** Minutes

Total Time: **40** Minutes

## INGREDIENTS

- ½ cup coconut flour
- 1 tablespoon psyllium husk
- 1 tablespoon ghee
- ½ tsp baking powder
- ½ tsp salt
- 1 cup boiling water

## DIRECTIONS

1. In a bowl mix all ingredients and refrigerate
2. Divine the dough into 6 balls
3. Heat a cast iron skillet over medium heat and place ice naan ball
4. Cook for 2-3 minutes remove and serve

# PEANUT BUTTER COOKIES

Serves:        *12*
Prep Time:     *10*  Minutes

Cook Time:     *30*  Minutes

Total Time:    *40*  Minutes

## INGREDIENTS

- 1 cup peanut butter
- 1 tsp vanilla
- 1 tsp baking powder
- ½ tsp salt
- ½ cup keto sweetener
- 1 egg

## DIRECTIONS

1. Preheat oven to 325 F
2. Cream together all ingredients
3. Refrigerate for 15-20 minutes
4. Roll dough into balls and place on a parchment paper
5. Bake for 12-15 minutes

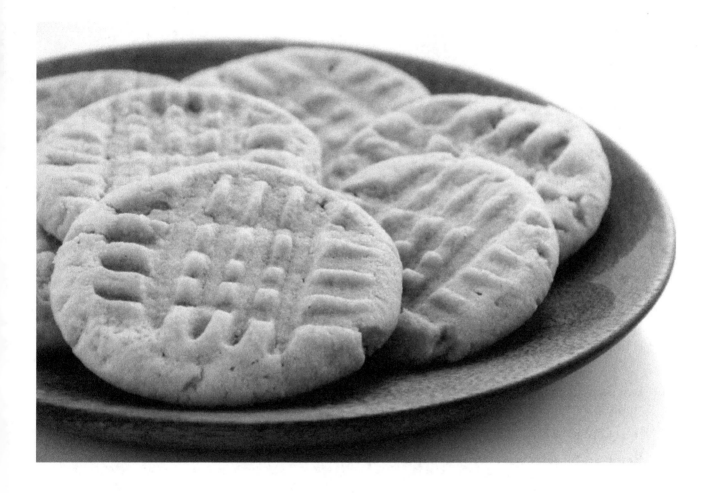

# BUTTERY KETO CREPES

Serves:        *2*

Prep Time:     *10*  Minutes

Cook Time:     *10*  Minutes

Total Time:    *20*  Minutes

## INGREDIENTS

- 3 eggs
- ½ tsp vanilla extract
- ½ tsp cinnamon
- 3 oz. cream cheese
- 2 tsp sweetener
- 2 tablespoons butter

## DIRECTIONS

1. In a blender place all the ingredients and blend until smooth
2. In a skillet pour batter and cook each crepe for 1-2 minutes per side or until ready
3. Remove and serve with berries, maple syrup or jam

# KETO LEMON FAT BOMB

Serves:        *4*

Prep Time:   *10*   Minutes

Cook Time:   *10*   Minutes

Total Time:   *20*   Minutes

## INGREDIENTS

- ½ cup coconut oil
- 3 tablespoons butter
- 3 oz. cream cheese
- 2 tsp lemon juice
- 2 tsp sugar substitute

## DIRECTIONS

1. Place all ingredients in a mixing bowl and mix thoroughly
2. Spoon 2 tablespoons into cupcake holders and freeze
3. Remove and serve

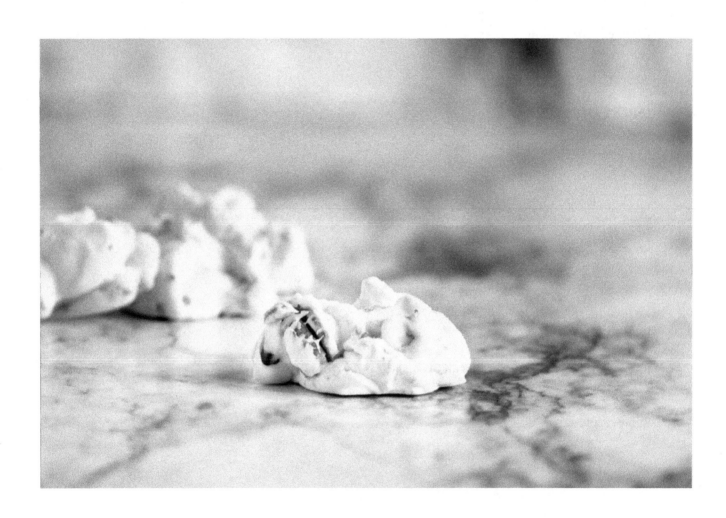

# PEANUT BUTTER BALLS

Serves:        *4*
Prep Time:     *10*   Minutes

Cook Time:     *30*   Minutes

Total Time:    *40*   Minutes

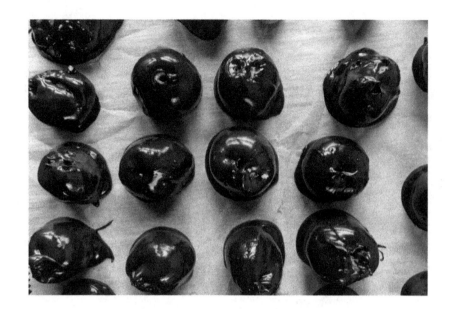

### INGREDIENTS

- 1 cup peanuts finely chopped

- 1 cup peanut butter

- 1 cup powdered sweetener

- 6 oz. sugar free chocolate chips

### DIRECTIONS

1. In a bowl mix peanut butter, sweetener, chopped peanuts, divide dough into 12 pieces and shape into balls and place on a wax paper

2. Melt chocolate and dip each peanut butter ball in the chocolate and place back on the wax paper

3. Refrigerate and serve

# NUT FREE KETO BROWNIE

Serves:           **8**
Prep Time:    **10**   Minutes

Cook Time:   **20**   Minutes

Total Time:   **30**   Minutes

## INGREDIENTS

- 5 eggs
- ¼ lb. butter
- 2 oz. cocoa
- ½ tsp baking powder
- 2 tsp vanilla
- ¼ lb. cream cheese
- 3 tablespoons sweetener of choice

## DIRECTIONS

1. Place all the ingredients in a lender and blend until smooth
2. Pour mixture into a baking dish
3. Bake at 325 F for 20 minutes
4. Remove slice into squares and serve

# SMOOTIES COFFEE SMOOTHIE

Serves:        *1*

Prep Time:     *5*   Minutes

Cook Time:     *5*   Minutes

Total Time:    *10*  Minutes

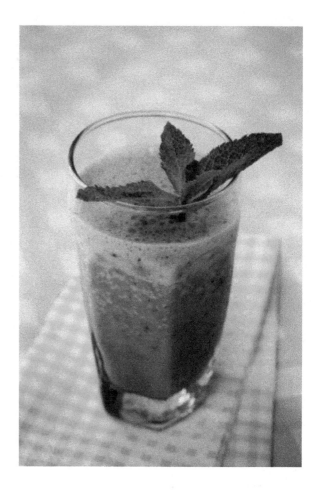

## INGREDIENTS

- 5 oz. cold coffee

- 3 oz. heavy cream

- 3 oz. almond milk

- 1 oz. sugar free chocolate syrup

- 1 oz. caramel syrup

- 1 tablespoon cocoa

- 12 oz. ice

## DIRECTIONS

1. In a blender place all the ingredients and blend until smooth

2. Pour in a glass and serve

# CHAI PUMPKIN SMOOTHIE

Serves: *1*

Prep Time: *5* Minutes

Cook Time: *5* Minutes

Total Time: *10* Minutes

## INGREDIENTS

- ¾ cup coconut milk
- 2 tablespoon pumpkin puree
- 1 tablespoon MCT oil
- 1 tsp chai tea
- 1 tsp alcohol free vanilla
- ½ tsp pumpkin pie spice
- ½ frozen avocado

## DIRECTIONS

1. In a blender place all the ingredients and blend until smooth
2. Pour in a glass and serve

# CASHEW SMOOTHIE

Serves:        *1*
Prep Time:    *5*  Minutes

Cook Time:    *5*  Minutes

Total Time:   *10*  Minutes

## INGREDIENTS

- 1 cup cashew mik
- 1 tablespoon keto MCT oil
- 1 tablespoon keto nut butter
- 1 tsp maca powder
- 1 handful ice

## DIRECTIONS

1. In a blender place all the ingredients and blend until smooth
2. Pour in a glass and serve

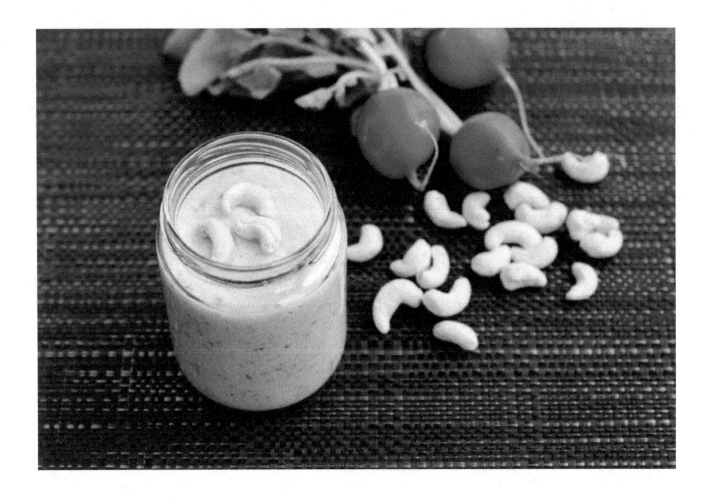

# BREAKFAST SMOOTHIE

Serves: **1**

Prep Time: **5** Minutes

Cook Time: **5** Minutes

Total Time: **10** Minutes

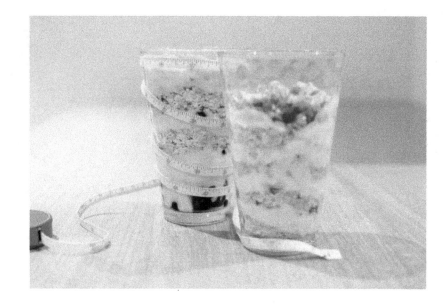

### INGREDIENTS

- ½ cup almond milk
- ½ cup coconut milk
- ½ coconut yoghurt
- ½ tsp stevia
- 3 strawberries

### DIRECTIONS

1. In a blender place all the ingredients and blend until smooth
2. Pour in a glass and serve

# KETO MILKSHAKE SMOOTHIE

Serves:        *1*
Prep Time:     *5*   Minutes
Cook Time:     *5*   Minutes

Total Time:   *10*   Minutes

## INGREDIENTS

- 6 oz. plain almond milk
- 3 oz. crushed ice
- 1 oz. heavy whipping cream
- 1 oz. raspberries
- ¾ oz. sweetener of choice
- ½ oz. cream cheese

## DIRECTIONS

1. In a blender place all the ingredients and blend until smooth
2. Pour in a glass and serve

# AVOCADO SMOOTHIE

Serves:       *1*
Prep Time:    *5*   Minutes
Cook Time:    *5*   Minutes

Total Time:   *10*  Minutes

## INGREDIENTS

- ½ avocado
- 2 tablespoons cocoa powder
- 2/3 cup coconut milk
- ½ cup crushed ice
- ½ cup water
- pinch of salt
- 1 tsp lime juice
- stevia

## DIRECTIONS

1. In a blender place all the ingredients and blend until smooth
2. Pour in a glass and serve

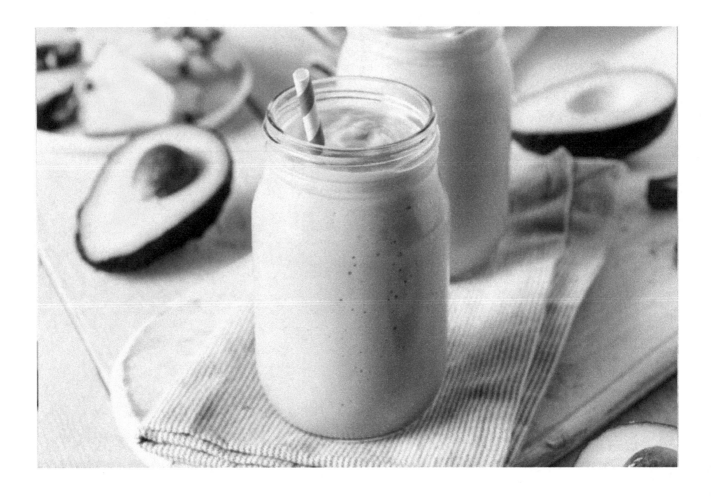

# COLLAGEN SMOOTHIE

Serves:         *1*
Prep Time:   *5*   Minutes
Cook Time:   *5*   Minutes

Total Time:  *10*  Minutes

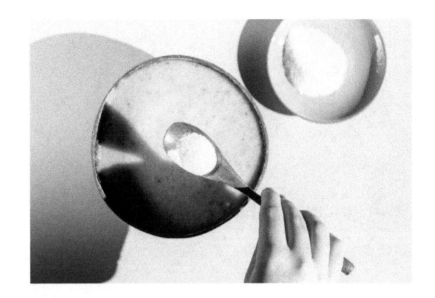

## INGREDIENTS

- 4 ice cubes
- ½ avocado
- 1 scoop keto chocolate collagen
- 1 tablespoon chia seeds
- 1 tablespoon almond butter
- ¾ cup heavy whipping cream
- 1 cup water

## DIRECTIONS

1. In a blender place all the ingredients and blend until smooth
2. Pour in a glass and serve

# FAT BOMB SMOOTHIE

Serves:        *1*
Prep Time:     *5*   Minutes

Cook Time:     *5*   Minutes

Total Time:    *10*  Minutes

## INGREDIENTS

- 2.5 oz avocado
- 1 scoop collagen
- 1 tablespoon cacao powder
- 1 cup almond milk
- 1 cup ice

## DIRECTIONS

1. In a blender place all the ingredients and blend until smooth
2. Pour in a glass and serve

# CINNAMON SMOOTHIE

Serves:        *1*

Prep Time:    *5*   Minutes

Cook Time:    *5*   Minutes

Total Time:   *10*  Minutes

## INGREDIENTS

- ½ cup coconut milk
- ½ cup water
- 2 ice cubes
- 1 tablespoon coconut oil
- ½ tsp cinnamon
- 1 tablespoon chia seeds
- ½ cup vanilla protein powder

## DIRECTIONS

1. In a blender place all the ingredients and blend until smooth
2. Pour in a glass and serve

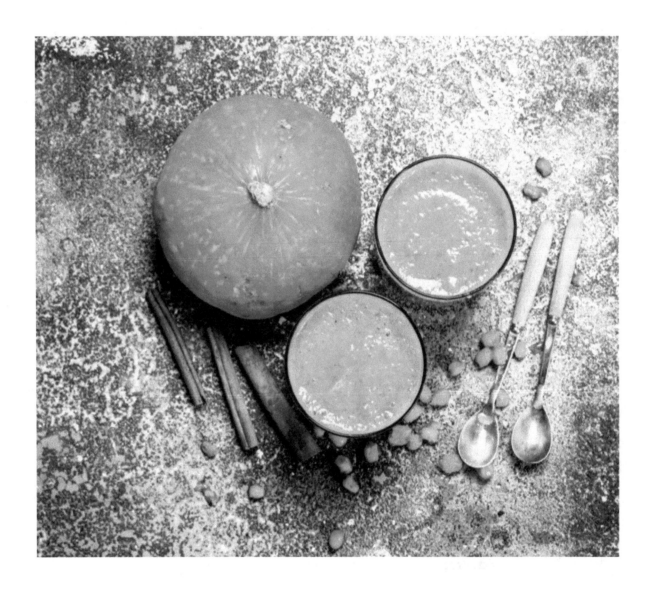

# TROPICAL SMOOTHIE

Serves: **1**
Prep Time: **5** Minutes

Cook Time: **5** Minutes

Total Time: **10** Minutes

## INGREDIENTS

- ½ tsp banana extract
- ½ tsp blueberry extract
- ½ tsp mango extract
- stevia
- 1 tablespoon oil
- ½ cup sour cream
- ice cubes
- ¾ cup coconut milk

## DIRECTIONS

1. In a blender place all the ingredients and blend until smooth
2. Pour in a glass and serve

9 781802 682960